Keto for Cancer

How to Use the Ketogenic Diet and Fasting to Fight and Prevent Cancer

<u>Disclaimer Notice:</u>

Please note the information contained within this document is for educational and entertainment purposes only. All effort has been executed to present accurate, up to date, and reliable, complete information. No warranties of any kind are declared or implied. Readers acknowledge that the author is not engaging in the rendering of legal, financial, medical or professional advice. The content within this book has been derived from various sources. Please consult a licensed professional before attempting any techniques outlined in this book.

By reading this document, the reader agrees that under no circumstances is the author responsible for any losses, direct or indirect, which are incurred as a result of the use of information contained within this document, including, but not limited to, — errors, omissions, or inaccuracies.

Table Of Contents

Introduction

Ketosis is a term many people might have heard, but few people understand what it actually means. Ketosis is a state in which the body burns fat to produce energy. Ketogenic refers to the process, or diet, in which ketosis is achieved.

Many celebrities have popularized the keto diet, as it is a great way to rapidly lose weight. However, there are many other reasons why a person might want to choose a ketogenic lifestyle. There have even been recent studies linking ketosis as possibly being a cancer reducer.

Ketone bodies are water-soluble molecules produced by ketosis, when the liver releases and burns fat or fatty acids for energy. Ketone bodies, ketones, ketogenic, and ketosis are all different terms with different meanings, but some people might have difficulty keeping up. The main thing to know is that it's all just about how the body processes food. The actual terminology can help in understanding a process better, but it isn't inherently necessary to actually live a ketogenic lifestyle.

Ketosis has a long history, as does most science. Ketosis is a state in which the body breaks down energy sources, so just like every other process in our bodies, it's been around for as long as we know. However, the history of how ketosis is studied is a lot younger. In just the past few decades, there has been more of an emphasis on ketosis as a way to cure, prevent, and treat cancer cells present in a patient's body.

The key thing to remember about ketosis is that it's all about fat. the body in ketosis finds a way to take fat cells and turn them into energy. This is why so many people have chosen this diet to help them lose a massive amount of weight rather rapidly. The reason why it's so popular is because not all the good food has to be given up. A ketogenic diet certainly isn't easy, but it still provides a dieter with plenty of options, so they don't so easily give up on their endeavors.

A ketogenic diet consists of eliminating as many carbs as possible, to less than five percent of a person's diet. Carbohydrates are in many different foods that plenty of people enjoy consuming. Foods like macaroni and cheese, cereal, donuts, and other delicious carb-filled foods are among some of the tastiest treats there are. Dieting is hard enough, so having to cut these foods from a meal plan can be challenging. A ketogenic diet still involves plenty of high-fat foods, such as bacon, cheese, and oils, allowing many people to still get the indulgent cravings that other diets don't offer.

There are many different variations of a ketogenic diet that a person might try. Some include cutting out meat completely, while others focus on only eating meat. Some people might try a ketogenic diet for a few months while other people have been dedicated to the diet for years at a time. That is what makes a ketogenic diet so great. It is adaptable and relatable for many different people.

One of the greatest things that has emerged surrounding a ketogenic diet is the idea that it might help lead to a reduction of cancer cells. The reason why we'll get into a little more later, but that idea alone has caused plenty of people to start a ketogenic diet.

A ketogenic diet is not something that's going to be right for everyone. Whether it's a health condition that already exists, or simply being a picky eater, there are going to be some people who just don't think that ketosis is what's going to help them reach their goals.

There are just as many people, however, who know that ketosis can be a life-changing state in their life that they would never have found if they didn't try something new and scary. No one whostarts ketosis finds it easy. The tastiest foods can be the most damaging to someone who wants to start a diet. Our stomachs can be much more powerful than our brains, so overcoming cravings and staying dedicated to a strict diet isn't something that everyone is going to do.

However, it's different when ketosis becomes a means to possibly cure, or at least prevent, cancer. It's not just about whether or not you'll be able to fit into a swimsuit at the beginning of summer. Those who look to a ketogenic diet as a cure are looking for help. They want to keep living, and they don't want the cancer to come back. When the stakes are so high, and potentially even deadly, of course, people are going to have a much simpler time sticking to a dedicated routine.

There is plenty of criticism around the ketogenic diet. Many people feel as though it's not safe, but this is likely just because there isn't enough research that supports it just yet. The idea of a ketogenic diet as anything more than just a way to lose weight is a relatively new concept. Fasting has been a common way for many cultures of all kinds to cure various health conditions.

A ketogenic diet is more of a response to fasting. Instead of the body having to starve itself in order to fight off certain diseases and conditions, ketosis allows a person to continue eating things they actually like while still producing the results that fasting might have on the body.

Ketosis is different on every single person's body, and the results will always vary from person to person. Everybody is unique, and the things you eat, and drink can affect everyone differently, no matter how similar the substances and regimens might be.

This book will cover everything to what the basis of a ketogenic diet is, to how a ketogenic diet can be achieved. I am not a doctor or a medical professional, so it is always best to seek that professional care before embarking on a journey towards a ketogenic diet. You might already be here because your doctor suggested starting a ketogenic diet, and that's great! This book will be just one of many resources that will help you on a path towards recovery and a healthier lifestyle overall.

Chapter 1 – Intro to Keto and Fasting

You might have first heard about a ketogenic diet from someone advertising products on Instagram. Maybe you heard about a friend or family member that managed to lose hundreds of pounds by starting a ketogenic diet. Or perhaps you know nothing about ketosis at all and this is the first time you are ever hearing about such an idea. No matter what your level of knowledge is, that's OK when starting a ketogenic diet. This book is going to take you through all the basics of ketosis and a ketogenic diet. By the end, you will be able to formulate your own specified diet plan that will help carry you through treatment, recover, and prevention of cancer.

The idea of keto is a diet primarily based around fats and avoiding carbohydrates as much as possible. A keto diet places emphasis on eating foods high in fats rather than ones loaded with carbs.

This doesn't mean eating fast food and just removing the fries and bun. There is still plenty of emphasis on choosing healthy foods.

There are many reasons why a person might choose a keto based diet. Whenever a person is looking to try a new diet, there are plenty of factors they should consider before following through. The most important one is finding something that suits an individual's lifestyle. A ketogenic diet might work for many people, but only those who are ready to commit to all of the challenges, and even risks, that a ketogenic diet might bring. One of the hardest parts about starting a ketogenic diet can also be having to give up carbohydrates.

Who doesn't love a big giant bowl of pasta? This can bring so much joy and happiness, but unfortunately, indulgences like this have to be avoided when starting a ketogenic diet. Through those carbs are absolutely delicious, they can also stop the body from achieving ketosis. The body works in very complex and mysterious ways. It's a tragedy that something so delicious can also be so bad for a person.

Carbohydrates provide a great amount of energy, but when the energy source comes from ketone bodies instead, there is a longer and consistent providence of energy. Imagine eating a huge bowl of pasta. Of course, that won't provide energy right away, and many people would pass out on the couch after stuffing their face with spaghetti. However, nay people choose to eat oats before workouts because of the great increase of energy that can come along with choosing the right kinds of carbohydrates.

Think of Thanksgiving. This holiday usually produces many people napping after they eat a large carb-filled meal. There was a myth for a long time that turkey is what caused many people to fall asleep after their big meal. That can be true, as turkey does contain chemicals that relate to drowsiness. However, most of the time, these bouts of napping occur because of all the carbohydrates consumed. Bread, pasta, potatoes, and high carb vegetables are staples at large Thanksgiving meals.

A ketogenic diet aims to make the energy come from a different source rather than carbohydrates. When this is done, that short and temporary bout of energy is diminished, along with the fatigue that can come along after a heavy carb meal. No matter how healthy a person might be or how much they exercise, a carb-heavy meal will still likely lead to a bout of fatigue at some point after consumption. A person seeking out a ketogenic diet might start with that reason alone to follow a new digestive path. This is just one of the many things that comes along with a ketogenic diet and needs to be remembered when thinking of why someone might choose this particular diet.

Simply put, ketosis allows for fat to be burned much faster than other diets. The main difference in a ketogenic diet is that fat becomes the main source of energy. Even people with low fat counts still have some that they could lose, and instead of the body needing high starchy foods filled with carbohydrates for energy, a ketogenic diet allows for a person's own fat to be used instead.

The downside, however, is that there must be a commitment to avoiding carbs. This can be a huge challenge for many people that decide to follow a ketogenic diet. Carbohydrates are obviously in starchy food and wheat-based products like bread, pasta, baked goods, potatoes, and anything else that has a high level of carbs. Besides just these obvious foods, sugary drinks, candy, and even many dairy and fruit products are full of unhealthy carbohydrates that a dedicated ketogenic dieter would need to avoid.

Foods like bacon, meat, and all the natural fats one could think of are welcome. That's one of the biggest draws of a ketogenic diet. Many people think that once they start going keto, they can eat as much bacon, salami, burgers, and other super fatty meats that they want. This is true for some people that choose a ketogenic diet but thinking like this can also be very dangerous.

These are the basic understandings of keto, ketogenic, and ketosis. Each of these terms is very different, and again, the reasons why a person might want to start a ketogenic diet are much different as well. losing weight and living a healthier lifestyle isn't the only reason a person might want to start a ketogenic diet either. Entering ketosis can also help with many other health issues, even including something as serious as curing cancer.

What is a Ketone?

Insulin helps the body regulate blood sugar. Everyone's insulin levels are different, and a person with diabetes might even need to take insulin shots to help regulate their blood sugar. Without any insulin, a person might get a high or low blood pressure, which can lead to very serious issues.

There are many different factors that go into what a person's insulin level might be, but it's true that it's made from mostly the same way in everyone's body. Insulin can come straight from sugar.

Sugar isn't just from candy, baked goods, or other sweets either. Insulin is necessary to help regulate the body's blood sugar, so one would assume that carbohydrates are necessary in order to ensure that they're getting as much insulin as possible.

When a person follows a high carbohydrate diet, they'll often find their body with large bursts of energy, but only momentarily. Loading up on carbs provides the body with energy, but once that source is depleted, the body will hit a low. This is why many people will feel very sleepy after indulging in a large bowl of pasta. Many people look to carbs for their workouts, but there will still likely be a bout of energy depletion once the carbohydrates are gone.

There is a lot of sugar in carbohydrates, so when the insulin struggles to regulate this sugar, it instead stores it as fat cells. The more sugary carbohydrates the person eats, the harder it will be for their body to maintain insulin levels. When the body is overloaded on bad carbs and sugars, they will accumulate fat cells much quicker than other healthier eaters. Not all carbohydrates are bad, and not all sugars can be dangerous either. The important part of consuming carbohydrates is ensuring that they will be productive to a lifestyle and not of causing more insulin to store the fat cells.

This is dangerous not only for those who want to avoid a high body fat, but for those who are diagnosed with cancer as well. Cancer cells have recently been shown to start eating off of glucose cells, which can directly come from carbohydrates. There is a general idea that fat cells will starve cancer, and glucose will feed cancer cells, which is the general idea of why someone would choose to start following a ketogenic diet.

The relation of sugar and cancer cells will be discussed later in the book. Since the body begins to store glucose as fat cells when more carbohydrates are taken in, some might wonder why they can't just eat carbohydrates for fat. The idea is that the cancer will eat off the carbohydrates and cause tumors to grow before they get the chance to turn into fat cells.

It's important first to understand this relationship to glucose, insulin, and sugar. Insulin is the body's regulatory hormone that keeps glucose in check. Glucose is derived from sugar cells, which can be very sneaky in certain carbohydrates. When you think of sugar and carbohydrates, they don't always seem to correlate. Carbs are associated with breads and pastas, and sugars are associated with sweets and junk food. There are actually a lot of both present in each of those categories.

Carbohydrates aren't bad. Many diets avoid them, but only because carbohydrates don't often aide in the burning of fat cells. Carbohydrates provide the body with an energy source. If there is no energy for the body to live off, it will not function properly. A ketogenic diet aims to give the body a source of energy other than carbohydrates in the hopes that more fat will be burned.

When the body is in ketosis, there are less carbohydrates present, less sugar. The goal of ketosis is to get the body to use a different source of energy that doesn't require carbohydrates. Lower levels of carbohydrate intake allow for less glucose in the body which can help to avoid creating more fat cells. A ketogenic diet chooses to eliminate carbohydrates completely in order to force the body to find a different source of energy. Instead of just limiting where the body gets its fuel, the body in ketosis forces the body's metabolism to completely shift its energy source.

In ketosis, the liver converts fats into ketone bodies. These become the energy source. When fat becomes the source of energy, it starts to get used up. This is great for those who want to lose massive amounts of weight. They can still eat a diet high in fat without worrying about gaining more weight.

Anyone is capable of getting to ketosis, but whether it's the right choice is something that should be seriously considered. Just as everyone's personality, beliefs, mindsets, and morals are different, so are their bodies. What works for one person doesn't work for others. Ketosis might come naturally to those whodon't eat many carbohydrates as it is. Others might struggle to find foods that they enjoy that don't involve carbs.

Some people might look to start a ketogenic diet by finding foods alreadyhigh in ketones, but that's not how it works. The goal of a ketogenic diet isn't to load up on ketones, but rather, force the body to produce more. There are a plethora of benefits that happen to the body once this happens, but it's important to understand what a ketone is first.

There are three types of Ketones:

1. Acetoacetate – this is the first ketone released when the body reaches ketosis. This is produced by the liver when glucose is not available. Fat is broken down into glycerol and fatty acid molecules.

2. Acetone - this is the least abundant ketone in the body, but when a ketogenic diet is started, it's the one that gets produced the most right away.

3. Beta-hydroxybutyrate – this eventually becomes the primary fuel.

Once ketosis is reached and maintained, these ketones will make up over 50% of the energy supply, as high as 70% for the brain.

History

Ketosis is a science, so it predates recorded history. Just like anything else a human body experiences, there isn't exact science known as to why our bodies do anything the way they do. Science isn't about finding the "why," however. There is more of a focus on studying how the body works the way it does. When it comes to the history of ketosis, it can be complicated. Ketosis is a form of fasting, and fasting has been around for as long as recorded history. Some decide to fast for religious purposes, and others do so in order to help make a bad health condition better.

Ketosis is a newer process, or at least, a newer idea in the science world. Within the past 50 years, ketosis has been studied more and more, and for reasons other than just how it can help the body lose a massive amount of weight.

A diet directed towards achieving ketosis is a result of a better solution needed for gaining the benefits of fasting. Fasting has plenty of benefits, but it's not easy. It's also not always safe. Doctors and scientists looked for a way that their patients could still eat and enjoy life while still reducing glucose levels and increasing their ketone bodies.

When the body is starved, it will turn towards fat cells as an energy source, which can be great for a number of reasons. The reduction of fat cells is good for anyone, not just for cosmetic reasons. Fat can become an energy source in ketosis. That's like finding a way to make garbage power your car! Fat serves a purpose and is still needed in everybody. However, an abundance is not recommended, so finding a way to put all that extra fat to use is a good thing.

This can also be incredibly dangerous, and though it might help a patient to lose weight or treat another disorder or disease, it could cause serious health issues that are worse than the original diagnosis. Some patients throughout history have found that a ketogenic diet has decreased their brain function, immune system, and muscle function.

Following a ketogenic diet allows a patient to still eat many foods they enjoy and provide their bodies with all of the things they need to live happily and healthy. The point of a ketogenic diet is to increase fat consumption, which can be found in some of the greatest foods. Ketogenic diets throughout history have been a response to a need for a solution better than fasting.

The main use of a ketogenic diet used to be in the treatment of children with epilepsy. Why this can work as a treatment is actually unknown to this day. It is only proven to work with those who experience seizures because research has proven that those who are in ketosis are less likely to have an attack. The specifics of why exactly this is the case is still fairly unknown to most medical professionals.

As more anticonvulsant medications came into play, the decision to follow this diet path decreased. This is because most kids aren't very good at monitoring their diet, and in order to be in ketosis, a strict regimen has to be followed. Going into ketosis isn't easy, and once it's reached, it can be even harder to maintain. This isn't easy for anyone, including children. Though anticonvulsant medications have allowed some children to avoid having to follow a ketogenic diet, there are still other benefits to this dietary path.

Fasting as a healing method goes all the way back to ancient Greece, when starving for weeks at a time was the best cure for patients with epilepsy. Even though ketosis has been around since then, there is still little known about why it produces the outcomes that it does. What is known, however, is that it works.

All About Fats

As research improved on the benefits of fasting, more was discovered about how the body uses fat when other energy sources aren't present. The body has to use something to get its energy, and when its main source is taken away – glucose – it will be forced to find something else to feed it. There are other energy sources the body could use, but it seems as though ketones are the greatest alternative.

Adding more fats to the diet would result in the body converting these into energy sources. Eating foods high in fat can sound scary. That's what many people are trying to avoid when they start dieting after all. When the body is using fat as an energy source, why not load the body with more of that source? It will only result in the body burning even more fat after all.

The point of ketosis is to get the body to use fats instead of carbs as a source of energy. This means avoiding high carb and sugary foods that might result in the body using glucose as energy and turning excess glucose into fat.

Fat can be a scary word for many people. Whether it's a way to describe someone, or just a description for an ingredient in a food, people have been scared by that three-letter word for decades. The reality is, however, that fat is good. Having too much of it can be a bad thing, but just like anything else in this life. Not all fat is bad, and fat is needed for everyone, not just those who want to achieve ketosis. While many people will spend their lives avoiding fat at all costs, ketosis is all about embracing that three-letter word. The more fat the better in a ketogenic diet, but as long as it's good fat, of course. There are different types of fats, and too much of the bad stuff can be life-threatening. Someone who wants to follow a ketogenic diet will soon understand just how crucial fats are in order to achieve their ketogenic goals.

What a Keto Diet Looks Like

Everyone's diet is different, and there is just as much variation with those who choose to follow a keto diet. There are many different types of ketogenic diets that different people might like to try. It can be very hard to find what kind of keto diet works best for an individual, so there is often a trial and error phase. Ketosis won't happen overnight, so it's important for many patients to understand that they will have to be patient when finding how to get their unique body into ketosis.

The main idea is a diet revolving around tons of high protein foods. This is usually found in a diet high in meat. Fatty proteins like bacon and pork can help elevate the fat intake of a person who wants to reach ketosis. Foods like ice cream, candy, and chocolate are high in fat, but they are also high in carbohydrates.

The only carbohydrates should be coming from fruits and vegetables. A ketogenic diet avoids many fruits as well because they are high in sugars, which in turn, means they're high in carbohydrates. A ketogenic diet is strict, but that by no means indicates that it will have to be boring. There are plenty of foods and recipes that include high fat foods without compromising too much in other areas that provide great flavor and interest.

Some people choose to cut dairy out, but others see the benefits of using the fats and sugars present in dairy. Dairy can also upset many adults, as most humans are supposed to follow a path of lactose intolerance. Though it's more common for people to eat dairy than to avoid it, there are plenty of health benefits to cutting dairy out of a ketogenic diet as well.

Some people think that you have to be wealthy in order to follow a ketogenic diet. Because it has recently been associated with different celebrities, many people assume that a ketogenic diet is unreachable unless you have the fortune that can come along with fame. That is not true at all. The opposite can be said, in fact. While having money is great when grocery shopping, there are still plenty of ways a person can budget and still buy food that helps them maintain ketosis. It's all about planning and being smart with their purchases. There are supplements and some higher quality foods that can definitely help and might cost more. Still, no one should be scared away from ketosis because they're afraid that they might not be able to follow through with the process.

Variations of a Keto Diet

Some patients find it difficult to give up carbohydrates. They are in everything that is good. Donuts, sandwiches, garlic bread, cake, cupcakes, cookies, and many more sweets and treats aresome of the greatest foods you might eat in a day. Unfortunately, these are all foods that should be avoided at all costs in a ketogenic diet, if made traditionally, that is. Even though some of the greatest foods can be dangerous for a ketogenic diet, there are still ways to incorporate ketogenic ideas into all diets.

Vegetarians and vegans aren't shy from achieving ketosis. Though meat is a huge part of many people on a path towards ketosis, a vegan doesn't have to compromise their beliefs just to get some protein. The same is said for vegetarians, who might even find that incorporating dairy is the greatest source of fat for their diets. Pescatarians know that fish is a healthier option than some heavier meats like beef or pork, but there are still plenty of fatty fish that can help a person reach ketosis.

As long as they can still find high protein foods, ketosis is achievable. This protein and fat can be found in dairy, legumes, beans, nuts, seeds, and many other vegetables. Legumes and beans can be tricky, however, because they are high carb, making them not keto. Some believe that following a vegan ketogenic diet is the greatest way to broaden one's pallet. Many patients are surprised at how many foods they can still eat even when they decide to cut out all meat and carbohydrates.

The Atkins diet is a notable ketosis diet, but only in the first stages. Many celebrities have taken to the Atkins diet as it is a healthy way to amass a great weight loss. There are still aspects of an Atkins diet that aren't fully ketogenic, however. For those who want to use ketogenic as a way to prevent or cure cancer instead of just losing weight might want to avoid the Atkins diet as their basis for reaching ketosis.

There are certain diets that can be altered to fit a person's lifestyle. Take veganism, for example. A vegan refuses to eat anything that comes from an animal. A vegetarian will have the same ideas, only they'll allow dairy and eggs back into their diet. Then comes in a pescatarian who allows fish into their meal plans as well. A plant-based diet can be very interchangeable depending on a person's lifestyle and what works best for them. A ketogenic diet can be altered the same way! It's mostly a variation of a low-carb diet, but everyone who practices ketosis can eat different meals and try new things that they might not have initially expected.

Exercise

Whether or not a person exercises while in ketosis is up to them. Exercise can help build muscle and reduce other parts of the body. This is something that can also be achieved through diet as well. The thing about exercise is that it takes up more of the body's energy. In order to provide proper nutrients, those in ketosis will have to eat much more when they're exercising, as they've already eliminated a major energy source.

Exercise doesn't always provide weight loss. Sometimes, it's just about toning the body and providing more muscle mass. Some find that exercise when in ketosis only leads to maintaining a certain BMI without providing any additional weight loss.

For someone with cancer, they might not have the energy to exercise. This is perfectly fine, and in fact, exercise isn't always encouraged. Having cancer puts the body through enough. On top of that, a ketogenic diet is a huge alteration in the body that can be exhausting as well. To exercise on top of that can put the body into overdrive, so it isn't always recommended to exercise if you have cancer and are in ketosis.

Ketosis allows for the body to still do what it's supposed to without having to sacrifice too much. It provides another energy source and allows for a way for the body to burn fat. Because this process is pretty effective on its own, not everyone that attempts a ketogenic diet has to exercise to see results. For those whoare disciplined in their dietary restrictions but don't have the energy to exercises, they might choose a path towards ketosis.

Exercise still helps. Exercise is never a bad thing, unless the active person is putting too much pressure on their body. The more a person exercises, the more their body can regulate their energy sources, so more fat can be burned; it's just about finding the right diet and exercise combination that works for an individual and unique body.

Again, if a ketogenic diet is something you're considering, it's important to speak to a doctor before embarking on an exercise routine. Many people might think they can come up with a great diet and exercise plan on their own, but they might not end up getting the results they want. This leads to discouragement and failure, which happens all too often for those who want to try a new diet plan. Talking to a doctor is important because they can give better insight into what a person might need in order to have a successful journey when dieting and exercising.

Ketosis

In a normal metabolism, carbohydrates are converted into glucose. These carbohydrates are the main energy source, which is why even though these starchy and sugary foods can be bad, they are necessary in a food pyramid. If they are not present, the body will look for another energy source. Those who choose to embark on a keto journey are aiming to force their body to use fat cells as the energy source.

When the body reaches a state of ketosis, there are fewer carbohydrates, so the liver instead turns fat into ketone bodies, resulting in the replacement of glucose. These ketone bodies come from the liver and cause the body to break down fat cells. Once broken down, these fat cells provide the body with the energy it needs for every other function.

This leads to a massive burning of fat in the person experiencing ketosis. Once there isn't much fat left in the body, then the person in ketosis will likely choose to continue to feed their body fat instead of reverting back to their old ways of using carbs as energy. Ketogenic diets don't have to last for life. The body is smart and will remember how to turn carbohydrates into energy should a person decide to take their system out of ketosis.

A person in ketosis has a better regulation of their blood. Too much glucose, or not enough, could cause high or low blood pressure. Both of these conditions can lead to even more health issues, some that go unnoticed. When a person is in ketosis, their glucose and insulin levels are much more regulated, allowing them to avoid an issue that might arise from having high or low blood pressure.

When the body is overloaded with fats, there will be less craving as well. Our bodies still crave fats, sugars, and carbohydrates. When we've provided our body with fat, and only fat as the energy source, we've given it what it wants, so cravings become reduced. This isn't the case for everyone, but many people in ketosis have reported that their cravings drastically reduce or become eliminated altogether.

Ketosis is how your body is choosing to get energy. It's not a fad, it's not a trendy diet, and it's not the solution to everyone's problems. It's a real process that body has gone through and isn't going away anytime soon. Some cultures even have histories of their people eating only ketogenic diets without them even being aware that this was a healthier alternative.

In order to reach ketosis, many believe that less than 5% of a diet should contain carbohydrates. Carbohydrates can't be completely avoided. There are going to be some carbs in every meal you have, and you should still be incorporating them into your diet. It's important, when trying to reach ketosis, that these carbs are kept at less than 1/20th of a person's diet.

When in ketosis, it has been discovered that an increase of ketones in the blood allows for a better appetite suppression. This is related to the reduction of cravings and allows people to not have to eat as much as often. Not only does ketosis help provide many people with a plethora of health benefits, but it can also help reduce a grocery budget as well!

If all that went over your head, don't worry. It's important to understand how a diet works so that it can be executed properly, but not everyone has a good grasp of basic science. What's most important to know is that ketosis is when the body uses fat as an energy source. It's as simple as that, and yes, it's as great as it sounds. Many people look to find an easy way to lose weight, a way that they can use their fat for good. Ketosis does just that. It's not easy for everyone especially those addicted to carbohydrates and sugar. Still, when the body enters ketosis, it can feel pretty incredible once the results start pouring in.

The Symptoms of Ketosis

The first symptom that the body might be in ketosis is bad breath. This is caused by the heightened number of acetones in the body. There isn't an exact reason why acetones cause bad breath, but many people in ketosis report that they might taste or smell of sulfur in the beginning stages of ketosis.

An increased level of energy and focus often surprises those in ketosis. The brain is no longer using glucose as an energy source, allowing for more clarity and focus. Having a healthy conscious mind always creates more clarity, and the more good foods the brain can eat, the better it will function.

The next stage will be weight loss. Even if exercise isn't a focus on someone's particular diet, weight loss will be reported. This is because the body is literally eating up a person's fat as a fuel source. What more could someone who wants to lose weight ask for? Well, maybe more macaroni and cheese.

Appetite suppression is likely with ketosis as well. Sugar can be incredibly addictive, so when a person avoids this as much as possible in their diet, they'll find that they'll end up having fewer cravings.

There are ways to test if the body is in ketosis. Kits and strips can be purchased online to help test if the body is in ketosis. These are important tools to help figure out if a person is following the right path or not. If someone has been on a ketogenic diet but they still haven't found their body to be in ketosis, there might be another underlying health issue.

Blood testing is the only accurate test for ketones, because urine strips only work in the beginning when you spill ketones in your urine. Once ketosis is established, you use the ketones for energy, so very little is left to spill in the urine. Checking your GKI is important throughout your ketogenic journey to ensure you remain in ketosis. This is especially crucial for fighting something as monumental as cancer. A formula for checking your GKI is in the next section.

Skin also improves for those who choose to try a ketogenic diet. When carbohydrates are avoided, along with sugary foods, the body will experience less inflammation. This will cause a reduction in acne or other health issues that the body might experience. A person's skin can really be affected by what they're eating.

Even if it feels like ketosis hasn't been reached, the body still might be in ketosis. Not everyone will experience all of the symptoms of ketosis, and that's okay. It doesn't work for everyone when it comes to weight loss, but it can be incredibly beneficial for those who want to reach ketosis as a solution for a different health issue.

When it comes to ketosis and cancer, some patients will find that their cancer cells stop growing once they've reached ketosis. Ketosis doesn't reverse cancer. It won't make the tumor disappear. When added to other treatments, however, the body in ketosis can reduce cancer symptoms and stop tumors from growing. The tumor can then be removed with radiation, chemotherapy, or surgery, and the patient will discover that the cancer does not grow back. These symptoms aren't immediate, and not everyone with cancer will find that ketosis works for them. This is still one of the most important symptoms when it comes to a person with cancer starting down a path towards ketosis.

GKI

You need to reach and maintain a certain GKI number to be in therapeutic ketosis, the extent of ketosis found to be effective for preventing and managing diseases like epilepsy, Alzheimer's, diabetes and cancer. GKI refers to a glucose keto index. These are what different levels of a GKI indicates: Anything less than 3 is high, 3-6 is moderate, and 6 or greater is low. The lower the GKI, the more benefits from ketosis. Your GKI can be measured by first measuring the glucose level in your blood. Then, write that number into this formula:

(Glucose Level / 18) / Ketones Level = GKI

Fasting During Ketosis

Sometimes, those in ketosis feel as though they hit a plateau. This is when fasting is considered. Fasting also might start at the beginning of a ketogenic diet. When the body is in a state of ketosis, it's basically reacting the way it would if it were in a state of fasting. The body knows how to adjust and store food when other energy sources aren't being properly provided. Fasting would be done if weight is no longer being lost and a person still has more pounds they want to shed. Instead of providing more energy sources to the body, fasting aims to force the body to use what it already has.

Fasting was the original reason many people opted for a ketogenic diet. Fasting is not easy. Humans are supposed to eat, like all animals. When that right is taken away, our bodies can go into panic modes. We can get grumpy, delirious, agitated, and delusional. However, our bodies are incredibly strong and can eventually adjust to fasting.

Ketosis and fasting can be used together. Someone might choose fasting as a way to get their body into ketosis. Once that has been reached, they can incorporate fats as the primary energy source. Fasting shouldn't be done for more than two days at a time. The body can react very negatively if fasting isn't carefully monitored. It's a dangerous approach to dieting and should only be considered after speaking to a professional.

It can be hard to partially fast or partially be in ketosis. When it comes to a ketogenic diet or one that involves fasting, it has to be all or nothing. There are some people who are "kind of" vegan, meaning they try to avoid meat, but might eat it now and again to avoid having to skip meals, or just to give into an intense craving. You can't be "kind of" in ketosis. You either are or aren't. Once a ketogenic diet is broken, the body can be pulled out of ketosis and the diet has to start over.

Ketosis is inherently a form of fasting. The idea started with trying to find a diet that could induce the symptoms of fasting without actually having to give up eating. Fasting and starvation need to be differentiated as well. A person who is starving is lacking what they need in order to survive. Someone who fasts should do so intentionally and in a controlled environment. You can't just decide to start fasting right now. There are steps that need to be taken before, during, and after a period of fasting to ensure that it's done safely and properly.

Choosing if Keto is Right

There are many reasons why a person might choose ketosis. A lot of people have looked towards a ketogenic diet as a way to reduce their weight. There are emerging health studies that prove that ketosis might also help alleviate other serious medical conditions. Losing weight is great, but when a diet can help treat other conditions, that is even better. The rest of the book will look at how ketosis might have a positive emerging relationship with the treatment of cancer.

Throughout the rest of the book, a more in-depth look will occur at the different benefits, purposes, and methods of ketosis. Before anyone decides to choose a ketogenic diet, it's always recommended that they speak with a health professional. Ketosis can be dangerous for some, and fasting isn't recommended for everyone. Someone with insulin deficiency might find that a ketogenic diet does the opposite of what it's supposed to do.

Here are some health conditions and other reasons why someone might choose to follow a ketogenic diet.

1. Epilepsy

2. Weight loss

3. Parkinson's disease

4. Multiple sclerosis

5. Alzheimer's disease

6. Fatty liver disease

7. Traumatic brain injury

8. Chronic migraine headaches

9. Autism

10. Polycystic ovary syndrome

The greatest way to determine if a ketogenic diet is right is to talk to a medical professional. It can be easy for different people to jump on the keto bandwagon, especially when they see gorgeous celebrities endorsing the diet on every media outlet they see. However, these people are not doctors. Even if your doctor doesn't suggest trying a ketogenic diet right away, they can still offer insight into what the personal risks might be for that one individual that decides to embark on a ketogenic journey.

Criticism of Keto

There are many people who have criticism of ketosis. Not all doctors will recommend ketosis for their patients, and that is because there is still plenty of research that needs to be done. While there is emerging proof that ketosis can change lives for the better, in some patients reducing cancer cells, a patient should still be very wary before choosing the path of ketosis.

The rest of the book will cover the benefits of ketosis, but it's important to understand the biggest reasons why someone might think that a ketogenic diet is not the right choice. There are studies that show the danger of ketosis, so it's really about an individual's circumstances when it comes to choosing if keto is right. The main criticisms are:

1. It's unhealthy – a high-fat diet has been linked to several other health conditions, so many are wary of embarking on a high-fat diet. However, most of this research has been conducted in situations where the participants were still taking in high levels of carbohydrates as well. A high-fat diet isn't dangerous if fat intake is the target, and other unhealthy sources are reduced.

2. It's not safe - some participants fear that embarking on a ketogenic diet isn't safe. They fear that their body might reach ketoacidosis, but this is a symptom that's normally seen in diabetic patients. There have been some reported instances of lowered brain function, fatigue, and other minor health ailments in those who have followed a ketogenic diet. It's important to remember that a strict ketogenic diet will likely help to avoid these negative symptoms.

3. It's not for everyone - this criticism is true. The ketogenic diet isn't for everyone, but that doesn't mean it can't still change the lives of many participants who want a healthier lifestyle than the unhealthy one they've grown accustomed to. What works for one person might be dangerous for another, but that doesn't mean that it should be avoided by everyone.

These criticisms are real and valid, but that doesn't mean that a ketogenic diet is wrong for everyone. There are certain people who find that a ketogenic diet is unhealthy for them, but there are plenty of others who completely turned their health around by cutting out carbohydrates. Some medical professionals believe that a ketogenic diet isn't safe, but there are a number of other professionals who would suggest this diet to their cancer patients. A ketogenic diet for sure isn't for everyone. Like any diet, there are certain criticisms and certain praises that exist around a ketogenic diet. It's all about finding the balance and doing the proper research to ensure that the right decision is being made on an individual level.

Chapter 2 – Ketosis and the Body

Everyone's body is different, so ketosis might not answer every patient's needs. There are some people that can find that their body is at it's best when ketosis is reached. There are other patients that have tried everything, and ketosis is the one thing that will work for them. Alternatively, there have been instances in which ketosis has been life-threatening, so it's really important to do as much research as possible before choosing this lifestyle.

Before getting into cancer, it's important to look at how ketosis affects the body. We've discussed that when the body is in ketosis, it will use fat as energy as opposed to carbohydrates. This should be well known by now, but how does that have an effect on the body? As a whole, we discussed some symptoms, but we're going to break the body down into important sections and study how ketosis might have different effects on different parts.

In this chapter, ketosis will be the main focus. This chapter will try to educate the readers on how a specific targeted area of the body might handle itself once ketosis in a patient is reached. Later on, there will be more of an emphasis on cancer. Ketosis and cancer are both very complex subjects, so it's important that a basic understanding of each individually is established first before looking at how the two interact. However, there will still be mention of various cancers in each section.

When building a new lifestyle, especially one that might involve a ketogenic diet, it's important to come up with specific goals. Throughout the rest of the book, note-taking is encouraged in order to help come up with a specified plan to begin ketosis.

What are the goals that one has while reading this book? Is it to lose weight while preventing cancer? Is it to cure cancer or reduce cancer cells in addition to other treatment methods?

These goals might include targeting specific areas as well. Some patients have cancer in one specific area. Others have cancer throughout their entire body. Everyone's situation is different, so taking notes is crucial in order to come up with a specified plan that will help meet the goals desired.

It's never too early to start cancer prevention. Everyone is susceptible to cancer no matter what lifestyle they choose to live. Some people are at a higher risk for cancer because of their genetics. Others might not know a single person in their family that has cancer. Cancer isn't going to be the cause of death for everyone, but it is certainly still a large threat to everyone no matter their race, age, or gender.

By trying to dodge cancer, other health ailments can be avoided as well. A ketogenic diet is ideal because it doesn't just aide in the prevention and reduction of cancer, but it helps in other areas of one's health as well. There isn't as much research done in ketosis as a prevention of cancer, rather, how ketosis affects patients that are already diagnosed.

Targeting Specific Areas

By this part in the book, there should be a basic understanding of ketosis and what that is. You don't have to have a medical license to understand how the body breaks down food to gain energy. It's something that not many people remember from elementary school, but the better understanding a person might have over their body, the better they can formulate a specific and targeted diet that works for them.

In this section, specific types of ketosis will be discussed, and how they might affect that certain area. Ketosis has a different effect on each and every part of the body. Our different organs and systems all have different purposes, so once their energy source is disrupted, of course, there are going to be some changes.

There will also be a discussion in the different areas about how cancer also affects these certain organs. Cancer in every patient is different, and cancer in every organ is different as well. There are no two circumstances that are alike, though there can certainly be some relations connected between various cases.

As the two are juxtaposed in this section, it can become much clearer how a ketogenic diet might help prevent, reduce, and in some cases even cure cancer. Not every section will be covered, just the most important and common organs affected by a ketogenic diet. It's important to remember that a ketogenic diet effects an individual in every single way. there likely isn't the body part that won't feel the effects of a ketogenic diet. Every part of your body will react differently, and how that relates to certain cancers differs as well. the next sections will cover the general idea based around that specific area, ketosis, and cancer. If you have a specific area that we didn't cover, be sure to do the proper research before embarking on a ketogenic journey.

Heart

The heart can be seen as the center of the body. The heart pumps blood throughout every other part of our entire body, playing a crucial role in each and every function that exists within us. the heart can seem so small compared to other organs, and yet, it holds so much power. Hearts can experience love, and hate, and an individual's heart can be very sensitive to both emotional and physical factors. We only have one heart, so it's important that we treat it right. Unfortunately, there are far too many health conditions that can negatively affect the heart.

Millions of people lose their lives every year to heart disease. It can affect even the healthiest of people that seem to have a great diet and exercise regimen. Smoking and other lifestyle choices can increase the chances of heart disease, but it can still affect anyone no matter what decisions they might make for their body.

Fat seems to be a big threat to the heart, and a ketosis diet is full of fat. When it comes to a person in ketosis, however, that fat turns into the energy source, so it doesn't affect the heart as negatively as it might in other diets. A ketogenic diet also aims to focus on healthy fats, not ones that will clog arteries or cause high cholesterol.

Surprisingly, ketosis will only end up helping out the heart. Low-carb diets optimize cholesterol intake and allow the heart to function as it would in other circumstances. Keto macros refer to the three nutrients your body needs while on a ketogenic diet. These include: fat (70-80% of a diet), protein (20-25%), carbs (5-10%). While that's much higher than other diets, it's still all about healthy fat, and not ones that would normally attack the heart.

The heart is a muscle, and it should be treated as such. In some cases, ketosis can break down the muscle, but only when enough fatty acids aren't present to be the fuel source. Fasting can seem scary to some people as it can break down muscle mass.

Adding a ketogenic diet instead of just fasting allows the protection of muscles and instead, targeting of fat cells.

Lungs

Our lungs provide us with the air that we breathe. This is such an important function in our body that we were actually given two of them! Our lungs can be the strongest organs in our bodies, but they can also be very sensitive to outside sources.

Lung cancer is much too common, and many people believe this is because of cigarette smokers. There are many reasons why a person might have lung cancer, and while causation is important for prevention, it's also crucial to look at how certain cancers can be treated instead of dwelling on the past. It can be easy for cancer patients, especially those diagnosed with lung cancer, to want to give up hope. They might feel too much regret and remorse over the decisions they have made, but ketosis provides hope. A hope that there is still a cure out there and a way for things to get better.

Since ketosis is all about the metabolic process and digestive system, it would be assumed it wouldn't play as much of a role when it comes to lung cancer. When a person chooses to embark on a healthier lifestyle, they are improving the overall quality of every aspect of their life.

Lung cancer is caused most often by smoking, though many non-smokers are still at risk of lung cancer based on other factors. The air we breathe in cities and other highly polluted areas could cause lung cancer as well, so even those with healthy diets might still be susceptible.

The greatest way a person in ketosis can improve their lungs is by including a rigorous exercise treatment as well. Sticking to only a ketogenic diet might not reduce or prevent lung cancer, but it can significantly increase overall health, which in turn, can help aid the lungs as well.

A person that chooses to start a ketogenic diet might want to increase their fat intake even more to provide an adequate amount of energy for exercise. When the lungs are worked out, along with the heart, overall function is improved, and the risk of cancer is reduced.

A lung cancer patient might not find the cure they want with ketosis, but there are certain benefits to this process. A diet that avoids high sugar and carbohydrates will help reduce the inflammation a patient experience. This can be crucial in preventing and reducing cancer cells in the lungs.

There hasn't been enough research done to prove that a high saturated fat intake will lead to negative cardiovascular effects. In most cases in which a threat was discovered, it was because carbohydrate intake wasn't reduced. You can't live healthily on a high fat and high carbohydrate diet. You have to make the choice between one or the other.

Heart disease, cancer, or other ailments can be caused by a number of factors. Some types can't be prevented or controlled no matter how much a patient might try. That doesn't mean that a ketogenic diet might not still help reduce symptoms or aide in other cancer treatments.

No matter what those might be, there's a good chance a ketogenic diet will still help improve those factors.

Brain

Is there anything more interesting in theentire human body than the brain? What's so enthralling about our brains is just how little is known about them. There is still so much that needs to be understood about why we think the way we do. What separates a brain of a human from a brain of another animal? What chemicals are involved that make us think the way we do, speak the things we do, and have the thoughts and feelings that we do? If the brain gets sick, so can everything else. The brain is the most responsible organ in the body, and no other organ has nearly as much pressure to maintain operation levels.

The brain is one of the trickiest organs, but does that come at much of a surprise? The brain itself holds the cure for cancer, though it just doesn't know it yet. Everything we know about the brain we learned by using a brain! It's pretty crazy if you really think about it. Because this is such an important organ, it also happens to be very sensitive. Little is known about how the brain works, so even less is known about how to treat it should something go wrong.

The brain is a very selfish organ, but it's allowed to be since it's working all day, nonstop. Even during sleep the brain is working harder than any other organ. It's constantly telling your other organs what to do, sending signals all the time. Imagine if your boss was working all day, 24/7, with no breaks. You would understand if they wanted to take all the food from the rest of the employees first!

Because it's so busy, pretty much all the time, there's no chance for it to store any of its energy. Hence why someone who might get hungry might quickly start to snap! Our other organs store energy sources so that if they have to, they have a backup if we can't feed them. For this reason, some might find that ketosis affects their brain negatively. This is usually reported only in the early stages of ketosis, when grogginess and grumpiness kick in. This negative side effect might also be due to a withdrawal of sugar, so more research needs to be done as to why someone might be grumpy at the beginning of ketosis.

There's a rather heated argument going on in the health community on what the best resource of energy for a brain might be. Like the rest of the body's organs, glucose is the preferred energy source. When that is gone, it turns to fat, thus triggering ketosis. The brain can still use ketones as an energy source, meaning that it will function just fine during ketosis.

Being just hangry is never fun, but things get serious when a brain reaches hypoglycemia. This is a condition in which blood glucose is low, causing a person's brain to be fatigued and disoriented. Hypoglycemia is dangerous and if suspected, treatment should be taken immediately. If the brain doesn't work, nothing else will properly either.

It seems, then, that a brain in ketosis might always be in a state of hypoglycemia. This isn't necessarily true, as carbohydrates won't be completely absent. The brain will likely take first dibs on any carbs that your body takes in, meaning that it'll be just fine in ketosis.

In terms of brain cancer, however, ketosis might be the best option in reducing the chance of cancer cell growth. The main reason for a ketogenic diet in the beginning was for the reduction of seizures. While there still needs to be more research done to help figure out the risks of a ketogenic diet, more and more research emerges that might give hope that ketosis is the answer for the reduction of brain tumors.

Systems

Aside from just how beneficial a keto diet can be on the body, there are other factors that make this lifestyle a good one to choose. There are plenty of toxins in foods that can cause cancer, and a keto diet makes a patient more conscious about what they're choosing to put in their food. Ketosis does wonders for different organs, and the same can be said about various systems in the body.

The body has several different kinds of systems. The endocrine system is the one that's most responsible for producing insulin and ketones. If this system becomes affected there's a chance that even ketosis won't help reduce the effects. This doesn't mean that an effort still shouldn't be made to overcome this sickness.

The reproductive system is another tricky one that we aren't going to cover in this section. Both of these systems have very little research done on them in terms of how they are affected by ketosis. We could make our own speculations, but as someone who isn't a medical professional, it's best to not make assumptions on how ketosis and these systems might work together. Instead, we are going to focus on systems that have a little more research involved.

Muscles

We have muscles in every part of our body. It might not feel that way, but you're using muscles to read this sentence right now. You use muscles to furrow your brow, to chew your food, and to even wipe your own butt. Like our brain, our muscles almost never stop working. Thinking of the stomach, the bladder, and other organs can be strange when comparing it to the nonstop muscular system. Try lying down or sitting without using any muscles. You might find that even in the most relaxed position, you are still using some form of muscle.

Ketosis plays the biggest role when it comes to muscles. Many people wonder how they can build muscles without the intake of carbohydrates. While it's much more challenging, it is still possible. Muscles might also be affected by ketosis during fasting.

If a person decides to fast, they might choose to just not eat anything at all. The body then turns to fat cells, but when those aren't present, muscle will be broken down as well.

Digestive System

Our digestive system is the most important one when it comes to dieting. What we choose to eat and how much we choose to consume will directly affect our digestive system. This is the part that will be the most affected by ketosis. Going into ketosis is something that is specifically targeted at the digestive system. It seems as though taking care of a digestive system is as simple as just eating and drinking, but it's so much more complex than just that. It involves an intricate system of figuring out what nutrients are needed in order to survive happily and healthily. Surprisingly, what we eat can directly affect every other organ and system in our body.

A keto diet might be low in fiber, which can affect the digestive system negatively. At first, many patients report diarrhea when starting a ketogenic diet. There might be other reasons why a person experiences digestive issues when starting a ketogenic diet, including:

1. An increase of artificial sweeteners

2. Decreased electrolytes

3. Decrease in fiber

Water weight is usually the first to go when starting a ketogenic diet. This might cause dehydration which can lead to serious digestive issues as well. It's crucial to maximize water intake when starting a ketogenic diet to make sure a digestive system stays in check.

Keto is also known for helping improve probiotics in patients that choose this diet.

Choosing a more consciously-safe diet is always helpful to the body, and a digestive system is likely the first to reap the benefits.

The Risks of Keto

Just like everything else in the world, there can be certain risks a person takes when they decide to embark on a ketogenic journey. It can be risky to go for a walk down the street or to get into a car. Everything has its own risks, just at different levels. A ketogenic diet can be risky because you're directly changing how the body is processing energy. Energy is important in making sure that everything continues to run smoothly, so of course, if this gets disturbed, so will everything else. Before choosing to attempt to reach ketosis, it's important for a person to consider every risk that might come along with a ketogenic diet.

There is still so little known about the long-term effects of ketosis that a diet such as this is very much still up for debate. Not enough research is put into this diet, especially in its relation to cancer. Many scientists and doctors believed that cancer was a genetic mutation for a while, so this new idea that it's a metabolic condition is something that needs to be further studied.

The main criticism of ketosis is that it's not safe. Some feel as though depleting the body of what it needs is never good, but what exactly the body needs are still inherently up for debate. Everyone's body is different, and no two people need the same thing. A ketogenic diet could be dangerous, but it could also help save someone else's life.

Not all health options are going to be safe. Some people choose to eliminate meat from their diet, but others need meat in order to have the proper amount of iron in their body. We can study what other people eat, and what other animals eat, in an attempt to figure out the perfect diet. The reality is there is no one diet. There is no one magical meal plan that will suit every single person. even if there were, there are too many picky eaters for a lifestyle like that to work anyway.

Keto is something that can be long term for everyone that tries this particular lifestyle. It can be a solution to more than one health issue at once. Keto can also be a quick solution to someone's problems, such as losing a massive amount of weight in a healthy way at first.

Chapter 3 – Keto as a Cure

This is why you're here. There are many keto books about how to start a new diet, and what tasty recipes you can make on a ketogenic diet. That's all important, but what's more important than losing weight is extending your life. Cancer is tricky. It's dangerous, it's deadly, it's ugly. Ketosis is great for many reasons, but more and more research shows that ketosis might be able to reduce, reverse, and prevent cancer cells in an individual that has been diagnosed.

There still needs to be more research done on the subject, but the results are already surprising experts. Before we can truly understand the correlation between ketosis and cancer, it's best to have a good knowledge of what cancer is. We all have basic ideas of cancer, even if you don't know anyone who has been diagnosed. It's a scary thing that could happen to anyone at any time. There is no exact cause and no known cure. All we know are things that can *possibly* prevent cancer, and *possibly* treat it.

What separates cancer cells from regular cells is the metabolic process in which they use energy. This alone is a direct indication that there could be a treatment for cancer based on diet. Since cancer grows in whichever part of the body it affects, you wouldn't assume that a diet could change cancer, especially if it's in the heart or lungs. However, our food is our source of life. If that is altered, of course it can change the life of the cells that exist inside of us.

When an alternative method is presented to fasting, such as ketosis, there is less of a chance of the body becoming much weaker. Fasting can have plenty of health benefits, but it can also seriously damage the body. It can cause dehydration, electrolyte depletion, and muscle reduction. When a diet such as ketosis is introduced, the same fasting results are there with less of the negative side effects.

Someone with cancer is already putting their body through a lot. Cancer disrupts every part of the body no matter where it chooses to take root. A ketogenic diet is very challenging for many participants as well, but the key is finding a plan that doesn't have to be debilitating. There is research that backs the idea that a ketogenic diet can reduce cancer. It's not going to work for everyone, but when a patient is desperate for an answer, keto might be there to help.

A person has to be sure that this diet is something that can be manageable, along with other cancer treatments. A ketogenic diet can disrupt an already disturbed body. There's no sense in putting the body through something if the results aren't guaranteed. However, there's no way to ensure that a diet or a treatment will work, so the risk is going to be there. With a ketogenic diet, those risks might be lessened.

Ketosis is also known for reducing oxidative stress. This can have a direct correlation to increased cancer cells. Though the two might not be correlated, it's still worth studying further if it means helping just one person reduce their cancer symptoms.

What is Known About Cancer

Compared to medicine 100 years ago, it seems as though we're incredibly advanced. There was a time where a woman couldn't even get a cesarean section without a very high likelihood that she was going to die. Now, many women choose to get c-sections because it works better for their birthing plans. This alone shows how far we've come.

Unfortunately, we still have just as far to go in terms of medical advancement. While our lifespans only continue to get longer, we still have yet to determine how to properly treat cancer. There are many methods that various patients have tried that have given them freedom from this life-threatening illness. Unfortunately, there are just as many people who have lost their lives to cancer after trying absolutely everything.

There are over one hundred types of cancer, and there are likely going to be more to be identified as medicine advances. Cancer is one of the most challenging conditions that takes the lives of way too many people. There are plenty of other diseases that are life threatening as well, but cancer is so tricky because there is no known cure. There are ways to reduce cells and help patients get into remission, but no one can just take a pill and feel assured that they don't have cancer anymore.

What differentiates cancer in various patients is the type of cell that becomes affected. Some patients have skin cancer, others might have a cancerous tumor on their brain. Some patients might find that the cancer has grown into their blood, and others might just simply have to get a lump removed from their stomach. Cancer is different every single time it appears, which is why it can be so challenging to pinpoint the root cause.

Cancer is when cells in the body begin dividing uncontrollably. These eventually form tumors. What causes this rapid divide is still unknown. If the cause of cancer was certain, it would be much easier to find a cure, though still unlikely. There are certain speculations of what might cause cancer, and some fear that they risk cancer with everything they do. Cancer cells exist in everyone, but when they form tumors is when things can start to get dangerous.

The tumors grow and begin to interfere with various bodily functions. Brain tumors can be challenging because they'll grow into the brain and reduce functions. Other types of cancers might block off certain organs, not allowing them to function properly. It's not the tumor itself that always kills someone, but what that tumor prevents.

Not every tumor might be dangerous. Sometimes, benign growths occur in a specific spot and can be easily removed. A growth on the skin, in the muscles, or even in the lungs has the potential to be completely removed, with the patient never experiencing any negative symptoms other than some slight discomfort.

When cancer cells become malignant, the cells move throughout the body and spread to different areas. This is when cancer can become deadly. In some cases, it takes decades for cancer to take over the body. In other instances, it can happen within weeks.

Cell invasion occurs when healthy tissue begins to become destroyed. This causes whichever function the cell had to be disrupted, which can lead to other serious medical conditions.

Metastasis is when a cancer cell grows so rapidly that it has spread to other parts of the body. This isn't certain for everyone that is diagnosed with cancer, but it can certainly affect many.

What causes cancer differs in every patient, and it still can't be said with certainty what a root reason a person might have cancer might be. In most mortality cases, the cause of death is rarely where the original tumor starts. It's clear that when death might be likely from cancer, it's because the cells have grown rapidly.

Cancer cells ignore signals from the body, which cause them to grow uncontrollably. They don't function like any other cell, which is another reason they are so hard to understand.

While it is still being studied as to what feeds a cancer cell, there is research favoring the idea that cancer feeds on sugar cells. When one chooses a ketogenic diet, they are doing their best to eliminate the sugar cells, thus eliminating the cancer food source.

Alternative Cures

Many scientists hope that they will be the ones to find the cure for cancer. It hasn't happened yet, so many people feel as though it will never be discovered.

Some think that the answer might lie in the bottom of the ocean, in some sort of chemical that exists only in rare coral. Others believe that the cure for cancer might lie within ourselves, such as in our umbilical cord or other substance. There are methods that have proven to help some cancer patients stop their cancer cells from growing and reach remission, but what works for one doesn't always work for the other.

The first step someone might take when they find cancer cells in their body is to remove the tumor. In some cases, a tumor can be removed allowing a patient to live a normal and healthy life. In other cases, the tumor might continue to grow back. It could be removed again, but that varies from patient to patient.

Sometimes, the removal of a tumor can't be easily done, so a cancer patient might opt for other treatments. Removing a tumor along with other treatments is another option for cancer patients. How someone chooses to attack their cancer will be different in every single patient.

Popular treatments are chemo or radiation therapy. The purpose of these treatments is to stop cell growth. With radiation therapy and a removal of a tumor, cancer patients can find themselves in remission, living long and happy lives after they are diagnosed.

These methods work by destroying the cancer cells in the body. In some cases, they can completely eliminate the cells. In others, they only shrink the cells in size in order to alleviate pain or pressure caused by the tumors.

Chemotherapy has worked for many, but there are also many negative side effects. Chemo doesn't just attack the bad, but also the good. This affects the hair, nails, and other continually growing cells in a person's body. That is why many people will lose their hair while undergoing chemotherapy.

A cancer patient also has to be strong to begin chemo or radiation in the first place. Chemotherapy attacks the body, weakening the immune system and causing an overall sickness. It could help in the end, but those going through chemotherapy don't have it easy.

Cancer and Metabolism

In the past few decades, there has been more of an emphasis on studying the metabolism of cancer patients. Cancer has been studied in many ways, including throughout genetics. Some scientists believe that cancer is all genetics, and whether or not you get cancer is determined by your genes alone.

Others think that cancer is only a result of our outside world, such as environmental factors. The truth is, just as there is no one cure for cancer, there is no one cause. More recently, science has shifted towards studying cancer as a metabolic condition rather than anything previously thought.

When determining how to destroy cancer, it's important to figure out how it grows. It's important to determine what cancer feeds on in order to figure out what needs to be taken away in order to starve the cells.

Otto Warburg was an important biologist that discovered cancer cells flourish when using glucose fermentation. The amino acid glutamine also helps to feed cancer. Both of these are often found in carbohydrates. Before Warburg's research, many people believed that cancer was a genetic disease.

Cancer cells have more insulin receptors than normal cells as well. These insulin receptors allow them to take in a higher rate of glucose, which can result in their rapid development.

Those with high blood sugar levels have the lowest survival rate among cancer patients. This is because they are feeding the cancer cells with various carbohydrates.

Fatty acids, on the other hand, provide no energy to cancer cells. This can cause the cancer cells to starve and stop multiplying. How bodies metabolize various energy sources is crucial in determining how cancer cells are fed.

Starving the Cancer

If you want to kill something, how might you do it? Drowning, fire, and starvation are all surefire ways for death. You can't drown your cancer cells, or else you risk harming other aspects. You can't just go and set yourself on fire, as that's clearly dangerous as well. Starving yourself doesn't seem like the greatest idea, but maybe that is the basis for how cancer cells can be overcome.

Some believe that a ketogenic diet is crucial in destroying cancer cells, as the body in ketosis removes the source of energy for carcinogenic cells. A ketogenic diet removes carbohydrates, and cancer cells love eating up carbs in the body. Just like they can be an energy source for us, carbohydrates can be very powerful cancer fuel.

When these carbohydrates are removed, so is the source for cancer cells' energy. This results in the starvation of the cancer cells.

This can't be true for all types of cancer, but there is more of an emphasis on how cancer cells can be starved. The ketogenic diet seems to be one surefire way to ensure that cancer cells aren't getting the glucose that they need to rapidly grow.

Starving the cancer cells can keep them from growing, but it's important to remember that this doesn't always mean it will make the existing cells disappear.

Reducing Insulin

Insulin is a hormone that greatly benefits the body. It helps metabolize sugar cells, so those who lack insulin might experience certain health problems. While insulin is important, it appears that it also might help contribute to the growth of cancer cells.

Reducing insulin might be an important step in starving the cancer cells. Higher insulin levels have been linked to metastatic cancer.

Eating foods that are higher in sugar cause the body to produce more insulin. When there is an excess of insulin in the body, that just means more food for the cancer.

Increasing Ketones

Cancer cells will eat up the insulin in someone's body for their energy. Luckily, cancer cells do not know how to use ketones for their fuel source. This means that when ketones are replaced instead of insulin, there is less of a fuel source for the cancer cells.

Ketones have actually been linked to helping melanoma cells grow more rapidly, so it's important to discuss this treatment with a doctor before a dedication is made.

Losing Cancer Cells in Ketosis

What's important to remember when it comes to ketosis as a treatment for cancer is that a ketogenic diet isn't going to make a tumor disappear. Perhaps one day a diet will be discovered that uses cancer cells as an energy source, but for now, we will have to rely on ketosis to use up all our fat for energy.

Cancer can be incredibly aggressive. Once sugar is taken away, a cancer patient might discover that their cancer cells stop growing completely. This is because cancer loves sugar. When the sugar is gone, the cancer doesn't have anything to eat anymore. This causes the cancer cells to starve. The other cells that already grew will remain, but they can be removed in other ways with surgery or radiation.

Sometimes, starving these cancer cells will aide in other treatments. When the body is in ketosis, they take away the cancer's ability to secrete necessary chemicals to continue growing.

Cancer Cells and Sugar

When a person eats carbohydrates, their body takes these fuel sources and turns them into blood glucose. When the body detects a high amount of blood glucose, it will signal the pancreas to release a higher level of insulin.

Insulin is released into the bloodstream in order to push glucose into cells. This is because the body is attempting to use those glucose cells as an energy source. Not only do cancer cells use this glucose as an energy source, but they thrive from this specific fuel.

The point isn't to necessarily eliminate sugar, as the body still needs insulin production to thrive. It's key to keep this process low in order to ensure that the cancer cells aren't getting fed.

Chapter 4 - Vegan Keto Diets

There are so many incredible foods in the world that can be consumed, so why would anyone want to cut any of them out?

Unfortunately, not everyone is capable of eating all the things their heart, or stomach, desires. Lactose intolerance, peanut allergies, and other sensitivities to different foods can cause someone to miss out on a lot in their life, without having any control. It can be frustrating to have a body that doesn't let you eat the foods that you want. So, some wonder why they would deliberately choose to cut certain foods out of their lives unless they have to.

What many people don't realize is how great they will feel after these foods have been removed from their diet. Some older adults don't even realize they're lactose intolerant until they stop eating diary. They might just think that having a messed up digestive system is a party of getting older.

A keto diet is a diet that eliminates carbohydrates. A vegan diet eliminates anything that isn't from a plant or the earth, such as mushrooms or other edible fungi. Those who choose to eat a vegan diet will avoid anything that comes from an animal. This can be surprising when really studied. Popular sodas like Coca-Cola aren't even vegan because they use sugar derived from animal products. Soda isn't OK in a keto diet anyway but choosing two very limiting diets can be very challenging.

A vegan or vegetarian keto diet might seem counterintuitive. Proteins derived from meat can be incredibly fatty while still providing nutritional protein to the dieter. If a diet eliminates anything processed from an animal and all foods that are high in carbohydrates, many people might be left wondering, what is left? There are even certain vegetables that aren't safe in a vegan and keto diet.

Although finding a vegan and keto diet that works might seem like a concept more complicated than finding a needle in a haystack, it can be done.

A vegan ketogenic diet is possible. The emphasis should still be put on foods with a high fat content. Fat is most commonly associated with animals, but fat can be found in many other foods. Fortunately, there are plenty of types of fat that exist that are both keto and a vegan friendly.

A regular vegan diet might still contain plenty of pasta, bread, and other carbohydrates as a source of energy. A keto diet would eliminate this, so where would the energy come from? Other fats exist in various oils, nuts, and vegetables that can help a person reach ketosis. Throughout the rest of this section, we will discuss the various types of food that someone on a vegan and keto diet might want to include in their pantry.

A vegan diet is not only environmentally conscious, but it can also help reduce the risk of many serious health conditions. On top of that, those who participate in vegan diets usually weigh less and have a greater overall health. Choosing a vegan diet can reduce the risk of almost all cancers, so adding a keto diet on top of that can only help make matters better.

A person might choose a vegan diet because they want to protect the environment. There are many ways in which the meat industry has negative and serious impacts on the world around us. Others also understand that eating meat can be incredibly inhumane and abusive towards animals.

Aside from moral beliefs, there are also health benefits to following a vegan lifestyle. Red meat has recently been linked to causing cancer, and processed meat has been classified as carcinogenic. Choosing vegan food also means going towards something more organic and less likely to be processed. This can help prevent cancer as most vegans avoid foods and products that could contain carcinogens.

Whether humans are supposed to be meat eaters, or whether we're natural herbivores might always be up for debate. Some think that our teeth indicate that we were born to eat meat. Others look at our ancestors and other primates and see that they didn't need to eat meat to survive. What we were wired to do might never be determined, but going forward, it's clear to see the health benefits a person gains when they decide to go vegan.

There are many doctors and dieticians that don't recommend a vegan keto diet, so it's important to consider all the consequences before choosing this path. While it's not recommended, there are still many people who follow veganism for religious or moral purposes, so they know they have options too.

Those that choose a vegan keto journey have to be careful with what they decide to use as their protein source. A lot of vegan meat products are also over processed, with hidden carbs and useless/potentially harmful chemicals, fillers and flavors. A vegan diet might also be lacking in vitamin A and B12, so many other deficiencies can crop up unless you take supplements for vitamins and iron, zinc, potassium, magnesium, among others.

Red Meat as a Carcinogen

Red meat is not to be demonized in this book, but it should be known that red meat isn't even the top recommended meat in keto diet. Fattier meats like fatty fish, chicken thighs and duck are preferred. Some mistake a keto diet as one filled with meat, but those that want to maintain a healthy ketosis need to be smart about their protein sources.

Within the past decade, the International Agency for Research on Cancer has classified processed meat as a carcinogen. A carcinogen is anything that has been linked to be a cause of cancer. This doesn't mean that someone who eats processed red meat is instantly going to get cancer. Instead, what is understood is that a high intake of processed red meat might be the causation of certain cancers, should someone be diagnosed.

The most commonly known carcinogen is usually understood to be cigarettes, or any form of radiation that can for sure be blamed for causing cancer. The idea that processed meat has become linked to the possibility of causing cancer can be pretty frightening for many consumers. Parents pack their kids' lunches with sandwiches and slices of processed deli meats. How many pepperonis have been consumed on different slices of pizza all around the world? Processed meat is a big part of many people's diets, so the idea that this could be a cancer-causing food can be frightening for many.

Foods like hot dogs, hamburgers, and other types of processed meats are staples in many societies. Someone who might eat organically can still eat these types of meats without subjecting themselves to the risk of cancer, as processed meats are what's carcinogenic.

Red meat includes:

- Pork

- Lamb

- Goat

- Beef

The safest way to cook meat is to put it in direct contact with the flame, such as on a grill or on a stovetop. When the meat is processed in a different way, especially in mass produced factories, the carcinogenic factor is increased. These are the ways that meats might be considered processed:

- Salting

- Curing

- Fermenting

- Smoking

The worst types of meats to eat for someone who wants to reduce their risk of cancer include deli meats, such as packaged lunch meat like ham or salami. Hot dogs, processed sausages, and other kinds of pre-packaged meats are also dangerous.

In order to avoid the risk of cancer at all, many people choose to follow a vegan keto path. Not only has the study of red meat caused alarm, but the population affected by cancer is concerning as well. There seems to be a rise of younger adults with colon cancer, and many people are starting to wonder if it's because of all the processed foods we've been fed throughout our lives. There isn't enough research to back this, but many are speculating that the processed foods we're eating are causing much more damage than we originally thought.

Vegan Keto Staples

Coconut products should become essential for those who want to follow a keto diet. When a vegan keto path is chosen, coconut products can provide a great amount of healthy fat. Be sure to know the difference between products that include full-fat coconut milk versus products that just include coconut flavor. These might include various flavors of coconut milk, coconut cream, and unsweetened coconut.

Oil is an essential fat for those who are eating keto. Oil can also provide a great source of fat for those who need it in their vegan diet. Fatty oils include olive oil, coconut oil, MCT oil, avocado oil, and nut oil. These can be used to cook with, added to smoothies, or simply eaten with a spoon in order to provide the patient with the proper amount of fat to fill their ketogenic diet.

Nuts and seeds provide the greatest protein source for vegans, and they also provide a great amount of fat for a vegan diet. Nuts that are the highest in fat include almonds, walnuts, macadamia nuts, and brazil nuts. Be sure when choosing nuts for a ketogenic diet that they aren't processed with too much salt or sugar. Salt can be really beneficial to both a keto and vegan diet, but only the right kind.

Another great staple that incorporates both oil and nuts, are various types of nut butter. This includes almond butter, sunflower butter, cashew butter, and of course, peanut butter. Someone who is choosing a vegan keto lifestyle might try to make their own butter as well. Experimenting with consistencies can be a fun way to find a fat source that a patient really likes.

Vegetables are key to vegans. That's why the words are so closely related. However, there are many vegetables that are still loaded with carbohydrates and other dangerous starches that could possibly prevent ketosis from occurring in the body. The greatest kinds of vegetables to eat are non-starchy ones, such as leafy greens, zucchini, cauliflower and broccoli, peppers, brussels sprouts, and mushrooms.

Alternative protein sources, such as tofu and tempeh, also offer incredible sources of fat and protein to those who are seeking a keto and vegan diet. Be wary of choosing tofu, as there have been some studies that link tofu to the potential of rising cancer, particularly in men. While the research isn't there to completely eliminate tofu as a source, someone who's very wary of carcinogens should do their research before using this as a protein source.

Organic and whole food stores offer many various vegan alternatives to common foods that are already popular among most family's shelves. Cutting dairy is essential to being vegan, but there are ways to still get the great flavors and fats that dairy provides. This can be done through "dairy alternatives," which might include coconut yogurt, cashew cheese, vegan butter, and other forms of cheeses that are plant based rather than derived from animal products.

Avocados are like ketogenic superfoods. These smooth green vegetables provide a great amount of healthy fat, and they can be used in so many recipes. Avocados can be expensive and don't last as long as other produce, but they provide one of the greatest sources of fats for keto vegans, right up there with coconuts.

Fruits can be filled with secret carbohydrates and sugars that many keto vegans wouldn't expect. Fruits are a large part of regular vegan diets, but keto vegans have to be a little more careful with the fruit they decide to consume. Berries are probably the best fruit group for keto vegans, as they contain less sugar than other fruits. They also provide a great number of antioxidants, which have their own beneficial properties not inherently related to a keto or vegan diet.

Aside from berries, fruits like lemons, limes, cranberries, olives, tomatoes, and watermelon are all fruits that contain sugar, but not too many carbohydrates. These can be eaten in moderation and should really be the biggest providers of sugar in a keto vegan diet.

When creating a vegan keto grocery list, many people worry that their food will be boring. Flavor doesn't always have to come from meat and other fats. Fresh herbs can be used in salads and pretty much every dish that can be made, and they fit perfectly in both keto and vegan diets. Lemon juice is another great healthy acid to use when cooking and flavoring, again providing no setbacks to a vegan or a keto diet.

While it may seem counterintuitive to have a vegan keto diet, many users would be surprised at just how well they can go together. When carbohydrates, meat, and dairy are cut from a diet, many people will want to run away as fast as they can. This lifestyle doesn't have to seem so scary!

Not only do these staples cause a healthier gut, but other benefits will emerge as well. Many vegans have nicer skin and hair because they're receiving the proper nutrients needed to have these healthier qualities. Vegans overall are happier, more energetic, and have clearer minds. Whether this is because they're more conscious of what they're eating, or because of the quality of food they take in is yet to be determined. There's a general consensus that being vegan is the healthier option.

Even someone who still wants to eat meat can benefit from the core values of veganism. Those who eat vegan put an emphasis on whole and organic foods. They avoid processed foods as often as possible and eat things that were consciously created. This should be done as often as possible for everyone, not just vegans. The better the food we put into our bodies, the better the outcome afterwards.

Foods to Avoid

Most foods for a vegan and a ketogenic diet will be the same. What differs in a vegan diet is that no eggs, fish, beef, or poultry are allowed. Anything that comes from an animal cannot be included in a vegan diet.

The rest of this section will cover other foods that vegan keto dieters should avoid. That can be tricky, because all of these things provide a great deal of protein to the dieter. The previous section covers some great foods to add to a pantry or a shopping list. The next section will also cover meat alternatives and other ways for keto vegans to get their protein. In this section, we'll go over what should be avoided by anyone who wants to live a vegan keto diet.

Any grain cannot be eaten in a keto vegan diet. "In moderation," is a generous phrase to use here, but some grains can be consumed in small amounts while still maintaining ketosis. This is highly discouraged, as it might just end up leading to uncontrollable cravings. Those in ketosis can still consume some carbohydrates, but very few. Sometimes, it is better to just avoid carbs altogether than trying to just sneak a bite or a taste of the indulgent foods we miss so dearly.

Most people find that cutting whole wheat breads, oats, corn, and quinoa from their diet is the easiest way to avoid falling back into old, non-keto habits. On a regular vegan diet, these things can be consumed, but they will keep the body from entering ketosis.

Any processed sugar needs to be avoided on a keto vegan diet. Many vegans know already how bad processed sugar is, and much processed sugar actually derives from animal products. Popular sodas like Coca-Cola use sugar that includes animal bone char. Many candies also include gelatin, which is another derivative animal product. Processed sugar should also be avoided in a keto diet, as it can be filled with carbohydrates. Cane sugar, white sugar, maple syrup, honey, agave, and any and all artificial sweeteners should be avoided on a keto vegan diet.

Giving up processed sugar can be almost impossible for some. What many people don't realize is just how addicted they are to sugar. even someone who avoids candy and other sweets might still get debilitating headaches when they removed all processed sugars from their diet. Many people also realize that after they have given up these sweets, how powerful they can be when they eat them again. Someone who might drink an iced coffee every day may decide to give up this habit when starting a ketogenic diet. Then eventually, they might treat themselves to that sugary drink. After just a week of giving up that added sugar, they'll realize just how sweet that was once they get another taste. It can be shocking to realize how numb we are to added sugar! The scariest part is that this sugar can also be the fuel for cancer cells.

Any and all potatoes, such as taro, yams, and sweet, should be avoided in a keto diet. These can be sources of protein for those who want to live a vegan lifestyle, but they are filled with sugars and carbohydrates that will prohibit the body from entering ketosis. There are alternatives to these potatoes, such as easily seasoned vegetables like cauliflower, or even tofu.

Black beans, chickpeas, and lentils can be great sources of proteins for vegans. Many vegans will find that they can replace most meats in any given recipe with the right amount of black beans and seasoning. Unfortunately, these types of legumes are not good for someone on a keto diet. They are filled with carbohydrates as well, which again, will stop the body from entering ketosis. They can still be consumed in moderation, like most other things in this section. It's important that they're only used as small sides or garnishes, and not the main source of protein in a meal. This high level of carbohydrates can mess up the body in ketosis.

Protein Replacements

When something is really good, there are bound to be plenty of imitators to follow. That can be said about any and all meat. If there's a type of meat, there's a good chance that a vegan has found a way to mimic this without having to actually use any animal product. There are certain mushrooms that can be used in place of other protein sources as well, with some even tasting exactly like chicken.

Many people fear a vegan or vegetarian diet because they love meat so much. Fortunately, there are plenty of meat alternatives that can taste the same, or better, then the meat that we're used to. Of course, if imitation bacon is put next to the real thing, it's going to be very simple to tell the difference. As time goes on, however, vegans will realize that they are still getting their cravings filled with the imitation meat that they are consuming.

Just because someone chooses to live a vegan keto lifestyle doesn't mean they have to give up on all the meat in their life. Instead, they can choose to replace meat with protein replacements. Meat alternatives include anything that can be flavored, cooked, or mixed into a recipe like meat would be without actually containing any element from an animal. This section will go over popular protein replacements that are both keto and vegan friendly.

Tofu is derivative of soybeans, containing a high amount of both protein and calcium. It can be used in pretty much anything, whether it's something sweet like a smoothie, or a meat replacement in a dish like "chicken" fried rice. Many people won't even notice the difference between tofu and real meat if cooked and seasoned properly. Marinating tofu is the best way to ensure that no flavor is being compromised. Tofu can work like a sponge, absorbing the flavor of whatever you want it to.

Tempeh is similar to tofu, but a little less popular. It's a fermented version of soy that has a bit more of a grainy texture than tofu. It's usually used when substituting ground beef. Tempeh tacos, and tempeh used in chili recipes is very common for keto vegans. Tempeh doesn't take on the flavor as well as tofu might, but it still provides a tasty alternative to meat for keto vegans.

We briefly touched on how some believe tofu might lead to other health issues and sometimes impotence in males, so it's best to do research before incorporating too much tofu in a diet. Some common health issues associated with tofu and tempeh include:

- fatigue

- cold sensitivity

- dry skin

- constipation

- unexpected weight gain

Many keto vegans eat plenty of soy products without experiencing any of the above, but there are also a number of individuals that can have a soy sensitivity. Using 100% organic tofu and tempeh is the best way to avoid any health issues that might come along with using soy.

Seitan is derived from wheat gluten, and most commonly made with soy sauce, tamari, ginger, garlic, and seaweed. Since it does contain gluten, it should be eaten in only small amounts, but it can still provide protein that a keto vegan might need. It is also much lower in fat than the other meat alternatives we discussed.

Many stores offer products that are "vegan" or "meat alternatives," but it's important for those who are seeking ketosis to be very careful with these products. Reading the packages and figuring out the ingredients is important in ensuring that no secret carbohydrates or sugars are snuck into the diet.

In order to prevent deficiencies in a vegan keto diet, it's also important that the dieter ensure they are getting a proper amount of B12 and Vitamin A. Aside from taking supplements, this can also be done by eating brainless bivalves like oysters and clams to get your recommended intake of B12.

Some other vegan keto sources of pro-vitamin A include:

- broccoli

- cauliflower

- spinach

- kale

Vegetarian Ketosis

A vegetarian keto diet will follow the same rules discussed in the previous sections, only more animal products can be incorporated into a diet. Foods like eggs, milk, cheese, and yogurt are all foods that a vegetarian would include in their diet. The main difference between a vegan and vegetarian is that vegetarians allow dairy back into their diet. This is the only form of animal products that they allow themselves to eat.

A vegetarian who wants to achieve ketosis will make sure that their total carbohydrate consumption is less than 35 grams per day. A vegetarian who doesn't care about ketosis might load up on carbs as a way to get energy, but this can't happen if ketosis is desired. Including elements of ketosis into a vegetarian's diet can actually only heighten the eating regimen already in place. many vegetarians will substitute meat dishes with starchy foods or those surrounding carbohydrates. This is a sneaky way vegetarians will continue to gain weight and live unhealthily.

The key for a vegetarian to reach ketosis is to eliminate all animal flesh from their diet as well as focusing on low carbohydrate vegetables. At least 70% of their calories should come from fat, which is a high amount for anyone. The same meat substitutions can be used for keto vegetarians, and the same fruits and vegetables should be consumed as well.

Many health professionals feel as though a vegetarian diet is the best option for everyone, and whether or not ketosis is added is up to the individual.

There is a big misconception about vegetarianism, however. Many people think that they can just give up meat and continue to eat everything else as they would.

What happens is that many vegetarians end up replacing meat with some sort of carbohydrate or other unhealthy dish. Instead of eating a burger with French fries, a vegetarian might just eat an entire plate of fries. Just like any other diet, there are aspects of vegan and vegetarianism that can be very unhealthy. The key is finding balance and sticking to a dedicated meal plan that incorporates all of the necessary nutrients and vitamins.

Pescatarian Ketosis

A pescatarian ketogenic diet will include everything that was discussed above, only pescatarians also incorporate fish into their diets. Fish are the only animals that pescatarians allow themselves to eat.

High fat fish like sardines and salmon are a great way to get omega-rich fatty acids. These can help kickstart the body into ketosis. Of all the diets discussed in the chapter, one that includes fatty fish is probably the greatest one. Avoiding red meat is always a good idea, especially processed meats that might be carcinogens.

Fish is still a great meat that can provide a massive amount of protein without including any other health risks.

Chapter 5 – Living a Keto Lifestyle

Living a life surrounding a ketogenic diet is much more than just the things a person eats. It's also important to ensure that every other aspect is accommodating to this lifestyle. That's the only way that it can be truly maintained. Someone who wants to embark on a ketogenic lifestyle should build a support system. If a caretaker is wanting to go vegan, they should encourage other members of the family to try and incorporate these healthy keto methods as well. Not everyone in a family should have to go keto, but the members of a household should still offer support, avoiding eating non-keto foods too much in front of those who are trying to stay disciplined.

It can be hard for anyone to start a new diet, especially someone suffering from cancer. A diet takes discipline, knowledge, understanding, and acceptance. Even if someone lives a life in which they have plenty of free time to devote to a diet, they might still struggle to maintain the discipline it takes to follow through with a diet.

A person with cancer will find it even harder to start a new diet. Especially when they are feeling weak, tired, and hopeless. Someone who might be struggling to stay alive might not have what it takes to start a ketogenic diet. This lifestyle can be reached, despite how hard it might seem to achieve a lifestyle such as this.

It's important to ask for help when starting a keto diet. This might mean finding a friend who can help cook meals and take you grocery shopping. It could also mean reaching out to someone online who is having similar struggles when it comes to a ketogenic diet. There are plenty of online communities that give cancer survivors and those still struggling the tools that they need in order to create a support system around them. You are not alone in your struggle, no matter how much it might feel like that.

It can be done. For some, it has to be done. Cancer is evil. It can take over someone's life and rob them of everything they have. Many people who struggle with cancer will look for ways they can reclaim their life. A diet is one way. While more research still needs to be done that backs a ketogenic diet as a cure for cancer, this is one way that many people have been able to overcome their diagnoses and live a much freer and more rewarding lifestyle through recovery.

There are certain core values that someone who seeks ketosis should have. everyone's diet and personal choices are different. No two cancer diagnoses are the same, and no two ketogenic diets are the same either. However, there are some core values that are important to remember when embarking on a ketogenic journey.

The first one is to stay dedicated. Ketosis can't be achieved by living the same life that you have been, either before or during your cancer diagnoses. Discipline and dedication are required to follow through with this life-changing diet.

The second value is knowledge. You must always be aware of the things that you're putting into your body and the ingredients that any food you're consuming might contain. The knowledge doesn't stop there, or with this book either.

The more information you have on a subject, the better you'll be able to craft a specified diet that caters to your specific needs. Especially in the medical world, new information is emerging over health, cancer, and diets every single day. it's important to keep up with these studies in order to ensure that nothing is missed. Sometimes, what we think we know might end up being wrong after the proper research has been conducted.

When reading various news articles and studies, it's also important to look at the facts and the sources, and not always the headlines. A news article titled, "Red Meat Causes Cancer," might scare many, but readers won't always click to read the actual study that tells them that it's only processed red meat. They also might not realize that it doesn't necessarily mean that it causes cancer. Rather, that it has just been classified as a carcinogen.

The third value is acceptance. You will have to accept the fact that it is time for a change. Clearly, nothing else is working, and so a ketogenic might be the solution you have been looking for. You also must accept that this might not be the absolute solution. There are plenty of other ways a person might be able to reach ketosis, and there are other options for treating cancer as well. Accept that the method that works best for you as an individual, and not one that was specifically made for someone else.

Ketosis won't be reached without dedication and commitment. It's not something that can be stopped and picked up later. It takes a few days for the body to stop being in ketosis, so one meal won't break a diet. However, you can't just eat a ketogenic diet one day and expect results the next. It takes time and patience, and not everyone is capable of giving this to their own personal diet.

It might just be the most challenging thing a person has done, especially for those addicted to carbohydrates. Many people have used food as a comfort source, and when they're experiencing something as challenging as cancer, they might want to use this food as a way to make themselves feel better. You must be stronger than your urges to indulge in the very things that might actually be making you sick.

Remember that sugar is addictive, so it might be overcoming addiction that is the challenging part for some people. There might be moments of withdrawal, if someone is used to eating a certain amount of sugar every day. Headaches can occur in the beginning as well, but they'll eventually go away. What's important is staying dedicated and strong enough to push through those endless cravings.

The main idea is to reduce carbohydrates as much as possible while upping the fat intake. We've given some various ways to do this throughout the book, but it's up to you now to formulate your own plan that will work best in fulfilling your needs.

For some, cutting dairy out is crucial. For others, this still provides an adequate amount of fatty acids that they need to reach ketosis.

Fasting

When the body reaches ketosis, fasting might be required in order to rebalance the diet. Our bodies do a pretty good job of getting used to certain things, and this can include ketosis. Sometimes, fasting can help reboot the body and get its focus back on eating fat cells.

Fasting can be beneficial for those with cancer. The human body wasn't built to eat all day, non-stop. For some, this is the way their metabolism has developed. Think of animals in the wild. Some animals only hunt at night, and this might be the only time they eat within a three-day period. Between those moments of eating, the body will begin to fast.

There was a time when humans might only eat once a day, or once every other day. This was depending on their hunting schedules. There have always been benefits seen in fasting, but there is more research being done to determine the health benefits fasting might have on cancer.

If the cancer has nothing to feed on, it will eventually begin to die. The exact thing that fuels cancer isn't always known, but it is seen that when glucose cells are removed, the cancer no longer has an energy source to feed and grow on.

Fasting isn't going to destroy the body. It's important to remember that fasting is much different than starvation. The specifics are still being studied, but there is a correlation with fasting and cancer cell reduction.

During Ketosis

Fasting is a way to help kickstart ketosis. Avoiding food might be a challenging part of starting a new diet, but it can really help to get a ketogenic diet off to a good start.

Some that choose a ketogenic diet might go through bouts of fasting in order to overcome a moment of plateau. Fasting at night is the greatest time, as this is when the body's metabolism is the slowest.

Vitamins

When following a ketogenic diet, there are certain vitamins that should be incorporated into a person's diet. If certain foods are given up, various vitamins might be lacking as well. There are many supplements that a person who wants to achieve ketosis might consider taking.

B vitamins are essential, even for people who don't want to follow a complete ketogenic diet. Vitamin D is another important vitamin that cannot be overlooked.

Protein Powder

This can help those trying to follow a vegan lifestyle or just anyone in general that wants to up their protein intake. Protein powder can be added to smoothies, shakes, and other meals that need a little more of a protein boost.

Nutritional yeast also has a cheesy flavor, which could be added instead of using a high-sugar cheese. Many people will mix nutritional yeast with vegetables or gluten-free pasta in order to give an artificial cheese flavor that is a better substitute than processed cheeses.

Dining Out

Some people avoid going out to eat because they don't think that they'd be able to find anything they could eat. A ketogenic diet is becoming a more popular lifestyle for many people across the world. With this emerging popularity, many menus offer low-carb options that might fit into a ketogenic diet. Don't be afraid or embarrassed to ask a server for an ingredients list, or at least a better understanding of what might be in a dish on a menu. It's important that dedication and commitment is still being maintained when someone chooses to dine out.

Many vegan and vegetarian options can be eaten in place of other foods that might have higher carbohydrate content. If someone is struggling to find a ketogenic option on a menu, they might decide to look to the vegan, vegetarian, or gluten free section of a menu in order to ensure they're avoiding processed foods that might be high in carbohydrates.

Most food can be eaten by just taking the bun away. If ordering a burger, just ask for no bun, or extra lettuce to create your own lettuce wrap.

Cravings will soon pass, but you can be stronger than your biggest craving. Most people in ketosis find their cravings go away after the first steps, so remember that it won't always be like that.

The Biggest Challenges

When trying a new lifestyle, it's best to be aware of the biggest challenges that you might face. The more prepared you are to face these issues, the less likely you'll have moments when you slip up.

Everyone struggles to maintain a diet, but a ketogenic diet, especially for someone with cancer, can be especially challenging. It's important to never give up on a path towards ketosis, as it can be hard to fall back into once good habits are broken. For people that follow ketogenic diets, these are the biggest challenges they face:

1. Social eating – resisting the urge to eat what others eat. Many people might find themselves at a pizza party or a birthday dinner, unable to control their own cravings.

2. Finding enough energy for a workout – many people find that a keto diet might make them more tired on certain days, or that they can't build muscle mass as fast as they might have used to.

3. Convenient eating – finding food that can be taken on the go, or food that doesn't require a lot of preparation.

4. Getting bored with what is eaten – many people on a ketogenic diet might find that they fall into patterns of eating the same thing over and over again. There isn't as much to experiment with in a keto diet as there is one with no limits, but that doesn't mean that it has to be boring.

Conclusion

Choosing to embark on a ketogenic diet will never be easy. It takes plenty of time, dedication, and commitment. There are going to be days when dieters want to slip up and give it all up just so they can eat a tasty meal. We have learned by now that is completely fine! A ketogenic diet allows for slip-ups every once in a while, but not on a regular basis.

There are still plenty of delicious foods that can be consumed on a ketogenic diet, so not everyone has to give up on the things that they love. Alternative foods might not taste as good, such as cauliflower rice versus white rice. They do, however, offer many more benefits. It's going to take some adjustment, so no one can expect that they'll get used to a keto diet overnight.

Even those who have been in ketosis for years will find that they still have days when they want to completely change their life. Just like anything else that takes time and patience, ketosis is a constant upward battle. It will be worth it in the end.

There needs to be more research done on ketogenic diets, but what has been conducted so far has proven to be a good basis for innovative healthcare in the future.

Ketosis isn't reached overnight, but once it is, it can seem like magic is occurring in one's body. They will start to rapidly lose weight, have healthier skin, and in some cases, even reduce cancer cells.

In this book we have learned

1. What Ketosis is

2. What cancer is

3. How removing sugar from a diet can reduce cancer growth

4. Different ways that a keto diet can be planned

5. The basic foods that should go into a ketogenic diet

Although it might seem like it could be very challenging, a vegan keto diet is a path many choose to take as well. The idea of combining these two diets is finding an extremely specific health regimen that includes only eating foods that are absolutely necessary for further development. A vegan keto diet strips food down to its core, only taking in things that will benefit the eater in the end. Though there are certain benefits to eating foods like donuts, such as a better mood, in the end, these types of comfort foods only offer temporary relief.

Processed red meat has already been classified as a carcinogen, and it's not going to be the last of its kind to emerge as a health risk. The more processed food is studied the more is realized about the damaging effects it can have on the individual who chooses to consume anything processed. A vegan keto diet aims to eliminate anything process and focus on organic and whole foods that won't cause any risk to the dieter's health.

Although it seems as though both would be counterintuitive, many people will find that a vegan keto diet can actually work rather well together. There are foods that everyone should attempt to avoid, not just those who are going into ketosis. Sugary foods and other items loaded with carbohydrates can be helpful in moderation, but overall, the health benefits of cutting down carbs is undeniable.

Not everyone has to follow a strict ketogenic diet to discover certain health benefits. Just taking some of the core values, such as cutting out refined sugar, can really help a person take their health to the next level. There isn't an exact timeline of when things have to start either. It can be taken day by day, week by week, or month by month. Maybe it just starts with giving up soda. After that has become an easy habit, the next step might be to eliminate candy. Once all the sweets are gone from a person's diet, they can start with removing pasta or bread.

The process of reaching ketosis can be taken slowly. Once it is reached, there are certain strips and other kits that help a person test to ensure that their body is in ketosis. Once their body is in ketosis, a strict diet has to be followed to maintain this metabolic process. Having an occasional non-keto meal here and there isn't going to ruin everything, but it's still important to stick to the diet so as to make everything else in life a little bit easier.

There is still more to be known about ketosis, cancer, and the digestive system, but these ideas encapsulate the basis for research that could potentially change the future of medicine.

In conclusion, ketosis is not for everyone. Every physical body is different, and everyone's mind is different as well. When planning a diet, both of these must be considered.

Not everyone thinks that they need to see a professional for creating a diet, but it can't hurt in the end. A professional is trained in studying the human body, so they will know what's best when it comes to crafting a specific diet. Although many people feel as though they have the answers they need for a well-crafted diet, a nutritionist or other medical expert is key in determining what diet is going to work best.

There are certain challenges that everyone faces when starting a ketogenic diet. Some people struggle with how others perceive them and might feel pressure to skip out on their diet in social settings. A ketogenic diet isn't just how you eat or what you choose to snack on. It's a lifestyle that requires dedication and commitment. It won't be achieved through processed food, the drive-thru, or the frozen section at the convenience store. It's not easy, but once a routine is established, it's something that everyone can maintain.

After reading this, you don't have to decide to become keto right now. Take a day, a week, or a month to think about it. It's an important decision and certainly not one that should be taken lightly. The health benefits are undeniable, but it's not something that everyone will find ease with. Do the research to determine whether or not this is the right path for you.

Everyone is different and it's important to talk to a doctor before embarking on a journey such as this. Although it's risky, the payoffs can end up saving your life.

References

The Truth About Cancer

Medical News Today

NCBI

Harvard Health Publishing

AACR Publications

www.ingramcontent.com/pod-product-compliance
Lightning Source LLC
Chambersburg PA
CBHW081735250726
48657CB00010B/3282